Childhood Depression: Its Causes and Ways to Overcome It

Written By
Rafik Seddik

Table of Contents

A. The role of parents and caregivers in supporting a child with depression 1. Communication and emotional expression within the family 2. Creating a safe and nurturing home environment

B. Schools and educators as pillars of support 1. Implementing mental health programs in schools 2. Encouraging open communication and fostering emotional intelligence

VIII. Therapeutic Approaches for Childhood Depression A. Cognitive Behavioral Therapy (CBT) for children

B. Play therapy and expressive arts therapy

C. Mindfulness and relaxation techniques for children

D. Family therapy and its benefits for the whole family

IX. Medication and Treatment Options

A. Considering antidepressant medication for children

B. Potential risks and benefits of medication in children

C. Integrative approaches to treatment

X. Nurturing Resilience and Emotional Well-being A. The role of physical activity and a healthy lifestyle B. Fostering positive relationships and social support C. Teaching resilience-building skills in children

XI. Prevention Strategies A. Early intervention and mental health screening programs B. Raising awareness of childhood depression and reducing stigma C. Collaborating with schools, communities, and healthcare professionals

XII. Real-life Success Stories A. Inspirational stories of children who have overcome depression B. Insights from parents, therapists, and experts

XIII. Conclusion

A. Recapitulation of the importance of addressing childhood depression

B. Empowering readers with knowledge and tools to support children's mental health

C. Encouragement to seek professional help and maintain hope for a brighter future

I. Introduction

A. Definition and understanding of childhood depression

Childhood depression, also known as pediatric depression or childhood major depressive disorder (MDD), is a mental health condition characterized by persistent feelings of sadness, hopelessness, and a lack of interest or pleasure in activities that were once enjoyable. Just like depression in adults, childhood depression is a serious and complex mood disorder that affects how a child feels, thinks, and behaves.

Key aspects of childhood depression include:

1. **Emotional Symptoms:** Children with depression often experience overwhelming feelings of sadness, tearfulness, and irritability. They may have frequent mood swings and find it difficult to experience joy or happiness.

2. **Physical Symptoms:** In addition to emotional changes, some physical symptoms may manifest, such as changes in appetite and sleep patterns. Children with depression may either experience significant weight loss or gain and have trouble falling asleep or sleeping too much.

3. **Cognitive Symptoms:** Depressed children may exhibit difficulties with concentration, memory, and decision-making. They may also have negative and self-critical thoughts about themselves, others, and the world around them.

4. **Loss of Interest:** A child with depression may lose interest in activities they previously enjoyed, withdraw from friends and family, and have a decreased motivation to engage in daily activities.

5. **Social Withdrawal:** Depressed children may withdraw from social interactions and prefer isolation. They may feel disconnected from their peers and have trouble maintaining

relationships.

6. **Fatigue and Low Energy:** Childhood depression can lead to persistent feelings of fatigue and a lack of energy, resulting in reduced participation in activities.

It is essential to differentiate between occasional sadness or mood swings, which are normal emotions, and the persistence and severity of depression symptoms that interfere with a child's daily life and functioning. Diagnosing childhood depression involves a comprehensive evaluation by a qualified mental health professional, such as a child psychologist or psychiatrist, who will consider the child's symptoms, behaviors, and emotional experiences.

Childhood depression can have severe consequences if left untreated. It can impact a child's academic performance, social relationships, and overall well-being. Early intervention and appropriate treatment, which may include therapy, counseling, and in some cases, medication, can significantly improve a child's quality of life and help them develop healthy coping strategies for managing emotions.

B. Importance of recognizing and addressing childhood depression

Recognizing and addressing childhood depression is of paramount importance for several reasons:

1. **Early Intervention and Prevention:** Identifying depression in children at an early stage allows for timely intervention and prevention of potential long-term negative effects on their mental health. Addressing depression early on can prevent it from becoming a chronic and more severe condition in adulthood.

2. **Improved Quality of Life:** Childhood is a crucial period for development and learning. Untreated depression can interfere with a child's social, emotional, and cognitive development, leading to academic difficulties, strained relationships, and a diminished overall quality of life.

3. **Academic Success:** Depression can hinder a child's ability to concentrate, learn, and perform well in school. Addressing the underlying causes of depression can improve a child's academic performance and foster a positive attitude towards learning.

4. **Emotional Well-being and Resilience:** Recognizing and addressing childhood depression helps children develop healthy coping skills and emotional resilience. Teaching them to manage their emotions can equip them to navigate life's challenges more effectively.

5. **Reducing the Stigma:** By acknowledging childhood depression and openly discussing mental health, we can reduce the stigma associated with seeking help. This can create a more supportive environment for children to express their feelings and emotions without fear of judgment.

6. **Preventing Self-harm and Suicidal Behavior:** In severe cases, untreated childhood depression can lead to self-harm and suicidal thoughts. By identifying and addressing depression early, we can prevent such tragic outcomes and provide appropriate support to at-risk children.

7. **Building Healthy Relationships:** Addressing depression can improve a child's ability to communicate effectively and engage in healthy relationships with peers, family members, and caregivers. Positive social interactions are crucial for a child's emotional well-being and development.

8. **Positive Parenting and Caregiving:** Recognizing childhood depression allows parents and caregivers to be more attuned to their child's emotional needs and provide the necessary support and understanding. This can strengthen the parent-child bond and create a nurturing home environment.

9. **Enhanced Mental Health Literacy:** Recognizing and addressing childhood depression helps parents, educators, and society at large become more aware of mental health issues in

children. This increased awareness can lead to better support systems and resources for affected children.

10. **Long-term Mental Health Outcomes:** Addressing childhood depression sets a positive trajectory for a child's mental health in the long term. Proper treatment and support can significantly improve a child's chances of leading a mentally healthy and fulfilling life as they grow into adulthood.

In conclusion, recognizing and addressing childhood depression is crucial for promoting healthy development, preventing long-term consequences, and fostering a society that values and supports mental health in children. Early intervention and compassionate care can make a significant difference in a child's well-being and future prospects.

C. Purpose of the book: exploring the causes and providing effective strategies for overcoming it

The purpose of the book "Childhood Depression: Its Causes and Ways to Overcome It" is to provide a comprehensive and insightful resource that delves into the multifaceted aspects of childhood depression. The book aims to achieve the following:

1. **Educate and Raise Awareness:** The book seeks to educate readers about childhood depression, its prevalence, and its impact on children's lives. By raising awareness about this mental health issue, it aims to reduce the stigma surrounding it and encourage open conversations about mental health in children.

2. **Understanding the Causes:** One of the primary goals of the book is to explore the various causes and risk factors associated with childhood depression. By understanding the underlying factors that contribute to depression in children, readers can gain valuable insights into how to identify and address these issues effectively.

3. **Identifying Signs and Symptoms:** The book will provide

guidance on recognizing the signs and symptoms of childhood depression. It empowers parents, educators, and caregivers to be vigilant and responsive to the emotional well-being of the children in their care.

4. **Evidence-Based Strategies for Overcoming Depression:** The book will present evidence-based therapeutic approaches and strategies for overcoming childhood depression. It will explore different treatment options, including psychotherapy, counseling, and medication, while emphasizing the importance of tailoring interventions to suit each child's unique needs.

5. **Building a Supportive Environment:** The book will emphasize the significance of creating a supportive and nurturing environment for children with depression. It will offer practical advice on how parents, teachers, and caregivers can provide emotional support, communicate effectively, and foster a sense of safety and understanding.

6. **Promoting Resilience and Coping Skills:** In addition to addressing depression directly, the book will focus on promoting resilience and coping skills in children. Readers will learn how to teach children healthy ways to manage stress, emotions, and challenging situations.

7. **Preventive Measures:** The book will highlight the importance of preventive measures to reduce the risk of childhood depression. It will discuss how early intervention, mental health screenings, and promoting positive mental health practices can help prevent the development of depression in vulnerable children.

8. **Real-Life Stories and Examples:** Incorporating real-life case studies and success stories of children who have overcome depression will provide inspiration and hope to readers. It will showcase the resilience and strength that children can exhibit

when provided with the right support and treatment.

9. **Empowerment and Resources:** By the end of the book, readers should feel empowered with knowledge and equipped with practical resources to address childhood depression effectively. It will include a list of relevant organizations, support groups, and additional reading materials to further assist readers in their journey to support children with depression.

Overall, the book aims to be a valuable and compassionate guide for parents, educators, mental health professionals, and anyone interested in understanding childhood depression and supporting children on their path to healing and emotional well-being.

II. The Prevalence and Impact of Childhood Depression

A. Statistics and data on childhood depression rates

As an AI language model, I don't have real-time access to current data beyond my last update in September 2021. However, I can provide you with some statistics and data on childhood depression rates up until that time:

1. **Prevalence:** Childhood depression is a significant mental health concern worldwide. According to the World Health Organization (WHO), it is estimated that approximately 10-20% of children and adolescents experience mental health disorders, including depression.
2. **Age Range:** Childhood depression can affect children of all ages, but it becomes more prevalent as children grow older. It can manifest in early childhood and peak during adolescence.
3. **Gender Differences:** Studies have shown that depression rates differ between genders during adolescence. Females tend to experience depression at higher rates than males during this period.
4. **Comorbidity:** Childhood depression often coexists with other mental health conditions, such as anxiety disorders, conduct disorders, and attention-deficit/hyperactivity disorder (ADHD).
5. **Impact on Academic Performance:** Childhood depression can have a significant impact on a child's academic performance and attendance at school. Children with depression may struggle with concentration and motivation, leading to lower grades and educational achievement.
6. **Long-term Effects:** Untreated childhood depression can have long-term consequences, including an increased risk of

developing depression or other mental health disorders in adulthood.

It is essential to note that the data may vary depending on the country, region, and research methodologies used. Additionally, mental health statistics are continuously evolving as more research is conducted and awareness increases.

For the most up-to-date statistics and data on childhood depression rates, I recommend referring to reputable sources such as the World Health Organization (WHO), the Centers for Disease Control and Prevention (CDC), or other national health organizations that conduct research on mental health in children and adolescents.

B. Short-term and long-term effects on a child's well-being and development

Short-term and long-term effects of childhood depression can significantly impact a child's well-being and development in various ways. Here are some of the key effects:

Short-term Effects:

1. **Emotional Distress:** Children with depression experience intense and persistent feelings of sadness, hopelessness, and irritability, leading to emotional distress and an overall negative mood.

2. **Social Withdrawal:** Depressed children may isolate themselves from friends and family, leading to feelings of loneliness and a decline in social interactions.

3. **Academic Impairment:** Depression can affect a child's ability to concentrate, learn, and perform well in school, resulting in lower academic achievement.

4. **Physical Symptoms:** Children with depression may experience changes in appetite, sleep disturbances, and physical complaints like headaches or stomachaches.

5. **Low Self-esteem:** Depressed children often have negative self-

perceptions and low self-esteem, leading to a lack of confidence in their abilities.

6. **Risk of Self-harm:** In severe cases, children with depression may be at risk of self-harm or suicidal thoughts, necessitating immediate intervention and support.

Long-term Effects:

1. **Chronic Depression:** If left untreated, childhood depression can become a chronic condition, leading to recurrent episodes of depression throughout adolescence and adulthood.

2. **Substance Abuse:** Depressed children may be at a higher risk of developing substance abuse issues as a coping mechanism for their emotional pain.

3. **Social and Relationship Challenges:** The social withdrawal and emotional difficulties associated with childhood depression can lead to challenges in forming and maintaining healthy relationships throughout life.

4. **Academic Underachievement:** Untreated depression can have long-term consequences on educational attainment, leading to lower educational and career achievements.

5. **Physical Health Consequences:** Long-term depression can impact physical health, contributing to conditions such as chronic stress-related disorders, cardiovascular problems, and compromised immune function.

6. **Increased Risk of Other Mental Health Disorders:** Childhood depression is often comorbid with other mental health conditions. If left untreated, it can increase the risk of developing other mental health disorders, such as anxiety, eating disorders, and personality disorders.

7. **Interference with Healthy Development:** Persistent depression during critical periods of development can interfere with emotional, cognitive, and social development, potentially

leading to long-lasting consequences.

It is essential to recognize and address childhood depression early to mitigate these short-term and long-term effects. Appropriate intervention, support, and treatment can significantly improve a child's well-being, development, and long-term mental health outcomes. Early identification and access to professional help are crucial in helping children overcome depression and thrive in their lives.

C. Social and academic implications of childhood depression Childhood depression can have significant social and academic implications for affected children. These implications can impact various aspects of their lives, both in their interactions with others and their educational performance. Here are some of the key social and academic implications of childhood depression:

Social Implications:

1. **Social Withdrawal:** Depressed children may withdraw from social interactions with peers and family members. They may feel disconnected and isolate themselves, leading to feelings of loneliness and isolation.

2. **Difficulty Forming Relationships:** Children with depression may struggle to form and maintain healthy relationships with their peers. They may have trouble relating to others, leading to challenges in making friends and building social support networks.

3. **Peer Rejection and Bullying:** Social withdrawal and low self-esteem associated with depression can make children more susceptible to peer rejection and bullying, exacerbating their emotional distress.

4. **Conflict in Relationships:** Depressed children may exhibit irritability and mood swings, leading to conflicts in their relationships with others. This can strain friendships and family dynamics.

5. **Impact on Family Relationships:** Childhood depression can also affect family relationships, causing stress and tension within the household due to the child's emotional struggles.
6. **Social Skill Deficits:** Depression can interfere with a child's ability to develop and practice social skills, such as communication, empathy, and conflict resolution.

Academic Implications:

1. **Academic Underachievement:** Depressed children may have difficulty concentrating, completing schoolwork, and maintaining focus in the classroom, leading to academic underachievement.
2. **Absenteeism:** Depression can lead to increased absenteeism from school due to emotional distress and physical symptoms like headaches or fatigue.
3. **Decreased Motivation:** Children with depression may lose interest in school activities and have reduced motivation to participate in class or complete assignments.
4. **Cognitive Impairments:** Depression can affect cognitive functions, such as memory and information processing, making it challenging for children to retain and absorb new information.
5. **Disruption in Learning Environment:** A child's emotional distress and behavioral challenges associated with depression can disrupt the learning environment for other students in the classroom.
6. **Impact on School Performance:** Academic difficulties and reduced engagement in school can lead to declining grades and hinder the child's overall educational progress.
7. **Limited Educational Opportunities:** Prolonged academic underachievement due to untreated depression can limit a child's future educational and career opportunities.

It is crucial to address childhood depression proactively to mitigate its social and academic implications. Providing appropriate support, therapy, and interventions can help children manage their emotions, improve their social skills, and excel academically. Collaboration between parents, educators, and mental health professionals is essential in creating a supportive and nurturing environment that promotes the overall well-being of children with depression.

III. Identifying Childhood Depression

A. Recognizing the signs and symptoms in young children

Recognizing the signs and symptoms of childhood depression in young children can be challenging since they may not always have the verbal skills to express their feelings clearly. However, being attentive to changes in their behavior, emotions, and physical well-being can help identify potential signs of depression. Here are some common signs and symptoms to watch for in young children:

1. **Persistent Sadness:** A young child with depression may exhibit prolonged periods of sadness, tearfulness, or an overall "down" mood that lasts for most of the day and occurs nearly every day.
2. **Loss of Interest:** Depressed children may lose interest in activities they once enjoyed, such as playing with toys, engaging in favorite games, or spending time with friends.
3. **Irritability:** Instead of expressing sadness, young children may display increased irritability, mood swings, and temper tantrums.
4. **Social Withdrawal:** Depressed children may become more withdrawn and avoid interacting with peers or family members. They may prefer to be alone rather than engaging in social activities.
5. **Changes in Sleep Patterns:** Depression can affect sleep in different ways. Young children may experience difficulties falling asleep, frequent night awakenings, or excessive sleepiness during the day.
6. **Changes in Appetite:** Depressed children may show changes in their eating habits, such as loss of appetite or overeating,

leading to weight loss or weight gain.

7. **Physical Complaints:** Young children may express their emotional distress through physical complaints, such as headaches, stomachaches, or other unexplained aches and pains.

8. **Lack of Energy:** Children with depression may exhibit a decrease in energy levels and seem more lethargic or tired than usual.

9. **Clinginess:** Some young children with depression may become excessively clingy and reluctant to separate from their parents or caregivers.

10. **Difficulty Concentrating:** Depression can interfere with a child's ability to focus and concentrate on tasks, leading to academic challenges and learning difficulties.

11. **Expressing Guilt or Worthlessness:** Depressed children may express feelings of guilt or worthlessness, even when they haven't done anything wrong.

12. **Regression:** Some young children may display regressive behaviors, such as bedwetting or thumb-sucking, which they had previously outgrown.

It is essential to remember that young children may not have the vocabulary to express their feelings of depression directly. As a result, parents, caregivers, and educators should observe changes in behavior, emotional patterns, and physical symptoms to detect potential signs of childhood depression. If any concerns arise, seeking a professional evaluation by a qualified mental health professional, such as a child psychologist or pediatrician, is essential for proper assessment and appropriate support. Early identification and intervention can significantly improve the child's well-being and emotional development.

B. Understanding how depression may manifest differently in children than in adults :

Understanding how depression may manifest differently in children than in adults is akin to unraveling the intricacies of the human psyche, where emotions weave a tapestry of unique experiences. Just as each child is a distinct constellation of dreams and aspirations, so too does childhood depression assume a distinct form, distinguishable from the shadowed hues of adult melancholy.

In children, depression's cloak may be woven with threads of innocence, concealing an internal turmoil that often eludes easy detection. Their world, viewed through the kaleidoscope of burgeoning emotions, can be as perplexing as it is enchanting. The language of depression, restrained by tender tongues, finds expression through nuanced shifts in behavior rather than articulate words. Forlorn whispers of sadness reverberate within their young hearts, seeking solace amid the cacophony of daily existence.

While adults may bear the weight of depression upon their shoulders like a burdened soul, children carry it in the sparkles of their eyes. Behind seemingly innocent smiles may linger a profound sadness that colors their world in muted shades. The once vibrant colors of play and laughter may fade into subdued tones, signaling a silent struggle that only keen observers can discern.

Unlike adults, who may openly verbalize their feelings of despair, children might bury their emotions beneath layers of imaginative play, their expressions veiled behind the masks of make-believe. As adults seek refuge in solitude to introspect, children may seek solace in the company of toys, imbuing them with the unspoken sentiments of their hearts.

Depression's palette may brush their lives with a stroke of regression, revealing behaviors reminiscent of earlier, more innocent stages. They may seek comfort in the familiar embrace of habits long outgrown, seeking sanctuary within the past as they grapple with the uncertainty of the present.

C. The role of parents, teachers, and caregivers in early detection

The role of parents, teachers, and caregivers in early detection of childhood depression is paramount in identifying and addressing this mental health condition at its nascent stages. These key individuals play a crucial role as frontline observers, nurturers, and advocates for children's well-being. By being vigilant and responsive to early warning signs, they can provide timely support and intervention, paving the way for a child's emotional healing and growth.

1. Observation and Awareness: Parents, teachers, and caregivers spend significant time with children and are thus well-positioned to observe changes in behavior, emotions, and social interactions. Being aware of the signs of childhood depression enables them to identify deviations from a child's typical patterns.

2. Open Communication: Encouraging open communication with children is vital. By establishing a safe and non-judgmental space, parents, teachers, and caregivers can invite children to share their feelings and experiences, fostering trust and emotional expression.

3. Recognizing Behavioral Changes: Early detection involves recognizing subtle shifts in behavior, such as increased irritability, changes in sleep patterns, decreased interest in activities, social withdrawal, or academic difficulties.

4. Noticing Emotional Cues: Emotional cues, like frequent tearfulness, expressions of hopelessness, or feelings of worthlessness, can provide insights into a child's emotional state and indicate possible depression.

5. Collaboration and Information Sharing: Parents, teachers, and caregivers should collaborate and share observations to form a comprehensive understanding of the child's well-being. Regularly exchanging information can help detect and address issues promptly.

6. Identifying Triggers and Stressors: Recognizing triggers or stressors that may contribute to a child's depression, such as academic pressures, family changes, or social challenges, can guide intervention strategies.

7. Creating Supportive Environments: Parents, teachers, and caregivers can contribute to a child's emotional well-being by creating nurturing and supportive environments at home and in school.

8. Seeking Professional Evaluation: If concerns persist, seeking a professional evaluation by a qualified mental health professional, such as a child psychologist or pediatrician, is essential for accurate diagnosis and tailored intervention.

9. Implementing Early Intervention: Early detection allows for prompt intervention, offering the child timely support and guidance to cope with depression effectively.

10. Encouraging Parental Involvement: In schools, involving parents in their child's academic and emotional progress fosters collaboration between home and school environments, increasing the likelihood of early detection.

11. Fostering Resilience: Parents, teachers, and caregivers can promote resilience in children by teaching coping skills and fostering a growth mindset, which helps children navigate challenges and setbacks.

12. Practicing Self-Care: Caring for children's mental health also involves taking care of the well-being of parents, teachers, and caregivers themselves. Self-care practices ensure they are emotionally equipped to support the child effectively.

By collectively assuming the role of vigilant observers and compassionate supporters, parents, teachers, and caregivers can make a profound impact on a child's life, empowering them to traverse the labyrinth of childhood depression with strength and hope. Early detection and proactive support lay the foundation for healing and growth, ensuring that each child embarks on a journey towards emotional well-being and resilience.

IV. Causes and Risk Factors

A. Biological factors and genetic predisposition:

Childhood depression is influenced by a complex interplay of biological, genetic, and environmental factors. Understanding the biological and genetic components of this mental health condition is crucial for comprehending its origins and potential risk factors. Here's an exploration of the biological factors and genetic predisposition of childhood depression:

1. Neurotransmitter Imbalance: One of the key biological factors associated with childhood depression is an imbalance in neurotransmitters, which are chemical messengers in the brain. Specifically, imbalances in serotonin, dopamine, and norepinephrine have been linked to depressive symptoms in children.

2. Brain Structure and Function: Studies have found differences in brain structure and function in children with depression compared to those without the condition. These differences involve areas of the brain responsible for regulating emotions, mood, and cognitive processing.

3. Genetics and Family History: There is a genetic component to childhood depression, with a higher risk for the condition among children with a family history of depression. Certain genes and genetic variations have been associated with an increased susceptibility to developing depression.

4. HPA Axis Dysregulation: The hypothalamic-pituitary-adrenal (HPA) axis, which regulates the body's response to stress, may be dysregulated in children with depression. This can lead to abnormal cortisol levels and heightened stress responses.

5. Inflammation and Immune System: Inflammatory processes in the body have been linked to depression, and research suggests that inflammation and immune system dysfunction may contribute to childhood depression.

6. Early Life Adversities: Adverse early life experiences, such as childhood trauma, neglect, or abuse, can affect brain development and increase the risk of depression in children. These experiences may influence gene expression and neural pathways related to mood regulation.

7. Hormonal Changes: Hormonal changes during puberty can also influence mood and may contribute to the onset of depression in adolescents.

8. Temperament and Behavioral Traits: Certain temperamental and behavioral traits, such as high levels of sensitivity, introversion, or shyness, may be associated with an increased vulnerability to developing depression.

9. Epigenetic Factors: Epigenetic mechanisms can modify gene expression without altering the underlying DNA sequence. Environmental factors, such as stress or early-life experiences, can influence epigenetic processes, potentially increasing the risk of depression.

It's essential to understand that while biological and genetic factors contribute to childhood depression, they do not act in isolation. Environmental factors, such as family dynamics, peer relationships, school stress, and socioeconomic status, also play significant roles in the development and course of childhood depression.

Research in this area is ongoing, and a comprehensive understanding of the interplay between biological, genetic, and environmental factors is essential for developing effective prevention and intervention strategies for childhood depression. Identifying the risk factors and mechanisms involved can pave the way for early identification and personalized treatment approaches that address the unique needs of each child facing this mental health challenge.

B. Environmental triggers and stressors:

1. Family dynamics and conflicts

Family dynamics and conflicts can significantly contribute to childhood depression, as the family serves as the primary social environment and support system for children. The interactions, relationships, and communication patterns within the family can profoundly impact a child's emotional well-being and mental health. Here's a detailed exploration of how family dynamics and conflicts can be a cause of childhood depression:

1. Parental Conflict: Frequent and intense conflicts between parents can create a tense and emotionally volatile atmosphere at home. Children are highly sensitive to their parents' emotional states, and witnessing unresolved conflicts can lead to feelings of anxiety, helplessness, and insecurity. Prolonged exposure to such stress can increase a child's risk of developing depression.

2. Family Dysfunction and Communication Patterns: Dysfunctional family dynamics, such as poor communication, lack of emotional support, or inadequate expression of emotions, can leave children feeling unheard, invalidated, or emotionally neglected. In such environments, children may struggle to articulate their feelings, leading to suppressed emotions and a sense of isolation.

3. Parental Depression and Mental Health Issues: Parents who experience depression or other mental health issues may find it challenging to provide emotional support and engage in positive parenting practices. This can lead to disruptions in the parent-child bond and impact the child's emotional development, increasing the child's vulnerability to depression.

4. High Parental Expectations and Pressures: Excessive academic or behavioral expectations placed on children by parents can lead to chronic stress and feelings of inadequacy. These pressures may create an environment where a child's self-worth becomes tied to their achievements, making them susceptible to depressive thoughts if they perceive themselves as falling short of expectations.

5. Parental Rejection or Neglect: Emotional neglect or rejection by parents can be deeply distressing for a child, leading to feelings of worthlessness, loneliness, and abandonment. These emotional wounds can leave lasting impacts on the child's self-esteem and emotional well-being.

6. Divorce or Family Transitions: Major family transitions, such as divorce, separation, or the arrival of a new sibling, can disrupt a child's sense of stability and security. Such changes may trigger feelings of loss, fear, and confusion, increasing the risk of depression.

7. Sibling Conflicts and Rivalry: Sibling conflicts, rivalry, or bullying can contribute to a hostile and unsupportive family environment. Children may internalize these negative experiences and develop feelings of sadness, anger, or resentment.

8. Lack of Emotional Expression and Suppression: In some families, the expression of emotions may be discouraged or stifled. Children may internalize their feelings rather than expressing them openly, which can lead to emotional repression and increase vulnerability to depression.

It is essential to recognize that family dynamics are complex and multifaceted, and not all conflicts or challenges within a family environment will lead to childhood depression. However, identifying and addressing unhealthy family dynamics can significantly contribute to a child's emotional well-being and prevent or mitigate the risk of depression.

Interventions may include family therapy, parent training, open communication, and providing children with a safe and supportive space to express their feelings and experiences. By nurturing healthy family relationships and creating a nurturing environment, parents and caregivers can positively impact a child's emotional development and reduce the risk of childhood depression.

2. Traumatic experiences and adverse childhood events Traumatic experiences and adverse childhood events (ACEs) can have a profound

and lasting impact on a child's mental and emotional well-being. ACEs are negative experiences that occur during childhood, and they encompass a wide range of adverse situations that can disrupt a child's sense of safety, security, and emotional stability. These experiences can significantly increase the risk of developing mental health issues, including depression, in both childhood and adulthood. Here are some common traumatic experiences and ACEs:

1. Physical Abuse: Physical abuse involves the intentional use of force that causes harm or injury to a child. It can include hitting, slapping, punching, or any other form of violence.

2. Emotional Abuse: Emotional abuse involves persistent patterns of negative treatment, such as verbal insults, humiliation, belittlement, and threats, which can profoundly affect a child's self-esteem and emotional well-being.

3. Sexual Abuse: Sexual abuse involves any form of sexual contact or exploitation imposed on a child. This traumatic experience can lead to severe psychological consequences and emotional distress.

4. Neglect: Neglect occurs when a child's basic needs, such as food, clothing, shelter, medical care, and emotional support, are consistently not met. Emotional neglect, in particular, can be damaging to a child's emotional development.

5. Parental Substance Abuse: Growing up in a household where a parent or caregiver struggles with substance abuse can expose children to instability, neglect, and unsafe environments.

6. Parental Mental Illness: Living with a parent who has untreated mental health issues can lead to emotional neglect, inconsistent caregiving, and exposure to challenging situations.

7. Domestic Violence: Witnessing domestic violence between parents or caregivers can be traumatizing for children and can create an environment of fear and instability.

8. Parental Incarceration: Having a parent incarcerated can lead to disruptions in family life, financial hardships, and feelings of abandonment or shame.

9. Loss of a Parent or Caregiver: The death or permanent absence of a parent or primary caregiver can lead to feelings of grief, loss, and emotional distress.

10. Community Violence: Exposure to community violence, such as shootings, gang activity, or crime, can be distressing for children and create feelings of fear and insecurity.

The cumulative effect of multiple ACEs can be particularly detrimental to a child's mental health and development. Childhood trauma can alter brain development, increase the risk of behavioral and emotional problems, and lead to a higher likelihood of mental health disorders, including depression, later in life.

Early identification and intervention are essential to mitigate the impact of traumatic experiences and ACEs on a child's well-being. Providing a supportive and nurturing environment, access to mental health resources, and opportunities for healing and resilience-building can help children cope with the effects of trauma and overcome adversity. By addressing trauma and providing appropriate support, caregivers and professionals can help children foster emotional strength and work towards healthier, brighter futures.

3. Academic pressures and school-related stress:

Academic pressures and school-related stress are significant contributors to childhood depression and can have far-reaching consequences on a child's mental and emotional well-being. The modern educational landscape places substantial emphasis on academic achievements and performance, which can lead to heightened stress levels among students. Here's an exploration of how academic pressures and school-related stress impact children's mental health:

1. High Expectations and Performance Pressure: Children may face high expectations from parents, teachers, and themselves to excel academically. The pressure to achieve top grades, participate in extracurricular activities, and secure a promising future can create stress and anxiety.

2. Rigorous Curriculum and Overloaded Schedules: A demanding curriculum, coupled with extracurricular commitments, can result in overwhelming schedules, leaving little time for relaxation, play, and self-care. This constant rush can lead to burnout and emotional exhaustion.

3. Fear of Failure and Perfectionism: The fear of failure and the pursuit of perfectionism can become detrimental to a child's mental health. The relentless pursuit of excellence can lead to self-criticism, low self-esteem, and a sense of inadequacy.

4. Standardized Testing and Performance Assessments: Standardized tests and performance assessments can induce test anxiety and feelings of pressure to perform well, leading to stress and sleep disturbances.

5. Social Comparison and Peer Pressure: Children may compare themselves to their peers, which can amplify feelings of competition and inadequacy. Peer pressure to conform to academic and social norms can also contribute to stress.

6. Bullying and School Environment: Bullying and negative school environments can create a hostile and unsupportive atmosphere for students, leading to increased stress and emotional distress.

7. Lack of Support and Resources: Limited access to academic support, tutoring, or resources can exacerbate feelings of academic pressure and hinder a child's ability to cope with school-related challenges.

8. Heavy Homework Load: Excessive homework and assignments can create time constraints and feelings of overwhelm, reducing a child's ability to engage in restorative activities outside of academics.

9. Teacher and Parental Expectations: Unrealistic or overly demanding expectations from teachers and parents can impact a child's self-perception and academic confidence.

10. Impact on Mental Health: Prolonged exposure to academic pressures and school-related stress can lead to mental health issues, such as anxiety, depression, and feelings of hopelessness.

Addressing academic pressures and school-related stress requires a holistic approach that involves educators, parents, and policymakers. Creating a balanced educational environment that prioritizes the well-being of students alongside academic achievements is essential. Strategies to support children's mental health in the educational setting include:

- Promoting open communication and providing a safe space for students to express their feelings and concerns.
- Implementing stress-reduction techniques, mindfulness practices, and relaxation exercises in the curriculum.
- Reducing unnecessary academic pressures and encouraging a growth mindset that values effort and progress over absolute achievement.
- Offering support services, counseling, and access to mental health resources within the school setting.
- Fostering a positive and supportive school culture that emphasizes kindness, inclusivity, and empathy.

By addressing academic pressures and school-related stress, we can create an educational environment that not only nurtures academic success but also fosters the emotional well-being and resilience of our children.

4. Peer relationships and social challenges

V. The Role of Technology and Social Media

A. Impact of screen time on childhood depression

B. Cyberbullying and its effects on mental health

C. Strategies for promoting healthy technology use in children

VI. Coping Mechanisms in Children

A. Understanding how children cope with depression

B. The importance of healthy coping strategies

C. Teaching children emotional regulation and problem-solving skills

VII. Building a Supportive Environment

A. The role of parents and caregivers in supporting a child with depression

1. Communication and emotional expression within the family

2. Creating a safe and nurturing home environment

B. Schools and educators as pillars of support

1. Implementing mental health programs in schools

2. Encouraging open communication and fostering emotional intelligence

VIII. Therapeutic Approaches for Childhood Depression

A. Cognitive Behavioral Therapy (CBT) for children:

Cognitive Behavioral Therapy (CBT) is a highly effective and evidence-based therapeutic approach used to help children and adolescents address a wide range of emotional and behavioral challenges. CBT focuses on identifying and changing negative thought patterns and behaviors, leading to positive changes in emotions and overall well-being. Here's an overview of how CBT is adapted for children:

1. Cognitive Restructuring: CBT helps children recognize and challenge negative or distorted thoughts and beliefs. Therapists work with children to identify unhelpful thought patterns and replace them with more realistic and positive ones. This process empowers children to reframe their perspective and develop healthier ways of thinking.

2. Behavioral Techniques: CBT involves teaching children coping skills and behavioral strategies to manage challenging situations effectively. Children may learn relaxation techniques, problem-solving skills, and assertiveness training to build resilience and confidence.

3. Age-Appropriate Language: Therapists use language and interventions tailored to the child's developmental level, making CBT accessible and engaging for children of different ages.

4. Play and Expressive Therapies: For younger children, play and expressive therapies are often integrated into CBT sessions. Play provides a natural way for children to express their emotions and work through their feelings in a safe and non-threatening environment.

5. Goal Setting: Children work with the therapist to set specific, achievable goals related to their emotional challenges. Breaking down larger goals into smaller, manageable steps helps children experience a sense of accomplishment as they progress.

6. Homework and Practice: CBT often involves assigning "homework" to children, which may include practicing new coping skills or challenging negative thoughts in real-life situations. This helps children generalize their learning and apply it outside the therapy setting.

7. Parental Involvement: Parental involvement is crucial in CBT for children. Parents are often included in therapy sessions or provided with guidance and support to reinforce the child's progress at home.

8. Coping with Emotions: CBT equips children with tools to manage and regulate their emotions effectively. Children learn to recognize their emotions, understand their triggers, and develop healthy ways of expressing and coping with their feelings.

9. Building Resilience: Through CBT, children learn to identify their strengths and build resilience to face challenges and setbacks. This helps them develop a positive outlook and greater confidence in handling life's difficulties.

10. Prevention of Relapse: CBT not only addresses current challenges but also helps children develop skills to prevent relapse in the future. Children learn to identify early warning signs and implement coping strategies to maintain emotional well-being.

CBT is adaptable and can address various issues, including anxiety, depression, behavioral problems, trauma, and more. The collaborative and goal-oriented nature of CBT makes it well-suited for children, as it empowers them to take an active role in their healing process and equips them with essential life skills for emotional well-being throughout their lives.

B. Play therapy and expressive arts therapy

Play therapy and expressive arts therapy are two therapeutic approaches commonly used to work with children and adolescents. Both methods utilize creative and non-verbal techniques to help children express their emotions, thoughts, and experiences in a safe and supportive environment. Here's an overview of each therapy:

Play Therapy: Play therapy is a form of psychotherapy that allows children to communicate and process their feelings, thoughts, and experiences through play and creative activities. It is based on the understanding that play is a natural and essential means of self-expression for children.

Key Elements of Play Therapy:

1. **Therapeutic Toys and Materials:** Play therapists provide a range of toys, art materials, and props to encourage imaginative play. These may include dolls, puppets, sand trays, drawing materials, and more.

2. **Non-Directive Approach:** Play therapy typically follows a non-directive approach, allowing the child to take the lead in play. The therapist observes and joins the child in their play, offering empathy and support.

3. **Emotional Expression:** Through play, children can express emotions, recreate scenarios, and work through difficult experiences in a symbolic way. This can help them gain insight into their feelings and develop coping strategies.

4. **Healing and Growth:** Play therapy provides a safe and non-threatening space for children to process trauma, resolve conflicts, and develop social and emotional skills. It promotes healing and supports healthy emotional development.

Expressive Arts Therapy: Expressive arts therapy encompasses various creative modalities, such as art, music, dance, drama, and writing, to facilitate self-expression and emotional healing. It allows children to communicate through different art forms, each offering unique benefits.

Key Elements of Expressive Arts Therapy:

1. **Multimodal Approach:** Expressive arts therapy uses a combination of art forms to provide children with diverse ways to express themselves creatively. Children can choose the

medium that resonates with them the most.

2. **Symbolic Expression:** The creative process allows children to symbolically express their thoughts, emotions, and experiences, even when they might find it challenging to verbalize their feelings.

3. **Mindfulness and Embodiment:** Engaging in expressive arts activities can promote mindfulness and help children connect with their bodies and emotions in a holistic way.

4. **Therapeutic Metaphors:** The use of metaphors in expressive arts therapy can help children gain insights into their experiences and emotions, facilitating emotional processing and growth.

Integration of Play and Expressive Arts Therapies: Therapists often integrate play and expressive arts techniques, tailoring the therapeutic approach to meet the unique needs of each child. By combining the benefits of both modalities, therapists can create a comprehensive and effective therapeutic experience that promotes self-awareness, emotional regulation, and positive change in children and adolescents.

C. Mindfulness and relaxation techniques for children

Mindfulness and relaxation techniques are valuable tools for children to cope with stress, manage emotions, and promote overall well-being. These practices help children become more present, develop self-awareness, and cultivate a sense of calm and balance. Here are some mindfulness and relaxation techniques suitable for children:

1. Mindful Breathing: Teach children to focus on their breath, guiding them to take deep breaths in through their nose and out through their mouth. Encourage them to notice the sensation of the breath and how it fills their lungs.

2. Body Scan: Guide children through a body scan exercise, where they pay attention to each part of their body, starting from their toes and moving up to their head. This helps them become aware of any tension or discomfort and encourages relaxation.

3. Mindful Listening: Have children close their eyes and listen attentively to the sounds around them, including sounds inside their body, like their heartbeat or breath. Encourage them to observe without judgment.

4. Guided Imagery: Lead children through guided imagery exercises, where they imagine peaceful and serene settings. This can help them visualize a safe place where they feel relaxed and happy.

5. Mindful Eating: Encourage children to eat mindfully, focusing on the taste, texture, and smell of the food. This helps them savor their meals and develop a deeper connection with their senses.

6. Progressive Muscle Relaxation: Teach children to tense and then relax different muscle groups in their bodies. This technique helps release physical tension and promotes relaxation.

7. Mindful Walking: Encourage children to walk mindfully, paying attention to the sensation of their feet touching the ground and the movement of their body as they walk.

8. Breathing Buddies: Have children lie down with a stuffed animal on their belly. Instruct them to watch how the toy rises and falls with each breath, helping them practice deep and calming breaths.

9. Mindful Coloring: Provide children with coloring sheets and crayons, inviting them to focus on the colors and movements as they fill the page with vibrant hues.

10. Gratitude Practice: Encourage children to express gratitude by writing or drawing things they are thankful for each day. This practice fosters a positive outlook and appreciation for the little joys in life.

It is essential to keep mindfulness and relaxation activities age-appropriate and engaging for children. Making these practices fun and accessible will encourage children to incorporate them into their daily lives. Consistent practice can lead to increased emotional regulation, reduced stress, and improved overall well-being for children as they learn to navigate life's challenges with a sense of mindfulness and inner calm.

D. Family therapy and its benefits for the whole family

Family therapy is a form of psychotherapy that involves working with the entire family unit to address and resolve interpersonal conflicts, communication issues, and emotional challenges. It aims to improve family dynamics, enhance communication, and promote a supportive and healthy family environment. Family therapy offers numerous benefits for the whole family, and here are some of them:

1. Improved Communication: Family therapy provides a safe and structured space for family members to express themselves openly and honestly. It encourages effective communication, active listening, and understanding each other's perspectives.

2. Strengthened Family Bonds: Through the therapeutic process, family members gain insights into each other's feelings, needs, and experiences. This fosters empathy and strengthens emotional connections among family members.

3. Resolution of Conflicts: Family therapy helps identify and address underlying conflicts within the family. The therapist facilitates productive discussions and problem-solving, leading to resolution and decreased tension.

4. Enhanced Coping Skills: Family therapy equips family members with coping strategies to manage stress, emotions, and challenging situations. These skills empower the family to navigate difficulties together effectively.

5. Increased Empathy and Support: As family members gain understanding and empathy for each other's struggles, they are better equipped to offer support and validation during times of difficulty.

6. Positive Parenting: Family therapy can help parents develop effective parenting strategies, promoting consistency, and improving parent-child relationships.

7. Healing from Trauma or Loss: Family therapy can be beneficial for families dealing with trauma, loss, or major life transitions. The therapeutic process aids in healing and supports the family through the grieving process.

8. Reducing Blame and Shame: In family therapy, the focus is on understanding the family's dynamics rather than assigning blame to individuals. This reduces feelings of shame and encourages a shared responsibility for positive change.

9. Building Resilience: Family therapy helps families build resilience by fostering adaptability and problem-solving skills. Resilient families are better prepared to face challenges and recover from setbacks.

10. Prevention of Recurrence: Family therapy not only addresses current issues but also equips the family with tools to prevent future conflicts and challenges from escalating.

11. Enhanced Emotional Well-being: As family members experience improvements in communication and emotional support, their overall emotional well-being is positively impacted.

12. Greater Self-Awareness: Family therapy encourages self-reflection and self-awareness in each family member, leading to personal growth and improved relationships.

Family therapy recognizes that individual family members' well-being is interconnected with the overall family system. By addressing the family's dynamics and relationships, therapy can create lasting positive changes and improve the quality of life for every member. The collaborative and supportive nature of family therapy offers a transformative experience that empowers families to thrive and grow together.

IX. Medication and Treatment Options

A. Considering antidepressant medication for children

The decision to consider antidepressant medication for children is a complex one that requires careful evaluation and consideration of various factors. While antidepressant medication can be effective in treating depression and other mood disorders in children, it should not be the first-line treatment option. Here are some important points to consider:

1. Severity of Depression: Antidepressant medication may be considered when a child's depression is severe, persistent, or significantly impacting their daily functioning and quality of life. In mild or moderate cases of depression, other therapeutic interventions, such as psychotherapy or family therapy, are often recommended as initial treatment.

2. Age and Developmental Stage: The age and developmental stage of the child are essential factors in deciding whether to consider antidepressant medication. Medication options may vary based on a child's age, as some antidepressants are approved for specific age groups.

3. Risk-Benefit Analysis: The potential benefits of antidepressant medication should be carefully weighed against the risks. Some antidepressants may have side effects and potential risks, especially in children and adolescents.

4. Comorbid Conditions: Antidepressants may be considered if the child has comorbid conditions, such as anxiety or obsessive-compulsive disorder, where medication can effectively treat multiple symptoms.

5. History of Treatment Response: If the child has not responded to other treatments, such as psychotherapy or counseling, antidepressant medication may be considered as an additional intervention.

6. Safety Monitoring: Close monitoring is crucial when a child is prescribed antidepressant medication. Regular follow-up with a pediatrician or child psychiatrist is essential to assess the child's response to the medication and monitor for any side effects.

7. Informed Consent: Before starting antidepressant medication, parents or caregivers should receive thorough information about the medication's potential benefits, risks, and side effects. Informed consent is critical in the decision-making process.

8. Collaboration with Mental Health Professionals: The decision to consider antidepressant medication should be made collaboratively with mental health professionals, such as child psychiatrists or pediatricians, who have expertise in treating children and adolescents with mood disorders.

9. Use in Combination with Psychotherapy: For best results, medication may be used in combination with evidence-based psychotherapy, such as cognitive-behavioral therapy (CBT) or interpersonal therapy (IPT).

10. Family Involvement and Support: The involvement and support of the child's family throughout the treatment process are essential for the child's well-being and treatment success.

It's essential to recognize that every child is unique, and the decision to consider antidepressant medication should be tailored to each individual's specific needs and circumstances. The goal is to find the most effective and appropriate treatment plan that supports the child's mental health and overall well-being. Regular communication and collaboration between parents, caregivers, and mental health professionals are vital to ensure the child's safety and progress during the treatment process.

B. Potential risks and benefits of medication in children

When considering medication for children, it is essential to carefully weigh the potential risks and benefits. Medications can be effective in treating various conditions, but they can also have side effects and potential risks, especially in young individuals. Here are some of the potential risks and benefits of medication in children:

Potential Benefits:

1. **Symptom Relief:** Medications can provide significant relief from symptoms associated with various medical and mental health conditions, including depression, anxiety, ADHD, and more.
2. **Improved Functioning:** By managing symptoms, medications can improve a child's overall functioning, academic performance, social interactions, and quality of life.
3. **Enhanced Quality of Life:** Effective medications can lead to a better quality of life, allowing children to engage in daily activities more comfortably and confidently.
4. **Treatment of Serious Conditions:** In some cases, medication may be necessary to treat serious medical or mental health conditions that can have a severe impact on a child's health and well-being.
5. **Supporting Other Interventions:** Medications can complement other treatments, such as psychotherapy or behavioral interventions, and enhance their effectiveness.

Potential Risks:

1. **Side Effects:** Medications can cause side effects, ranging from mild to severe, which can impact a child's physical and emotional well-being.
2. **Long-Term Effects:** Some medications may have long-term effects that are not fully understood, especially when used in developing children.
3. **Risk of Dependency:** Certain medications may carry a risk of dependency or withdrawal symptoms if not carefully managed.
4. **Individual Variability:** Children can respond differently to medications, and finding the right medication and dosage may involve trial and error.
5. **Interactions and Safety Concerns:** Some medications may interact with other drugs or medical conditions, leading to

potential safety concerns.

6. **Stigmatization:** Taking medication may lead to stigmatization or negative perceptions from peers or society.
7. **Ethical Considerations:** There are ethical considerations related to medicating children, particularly when the child's preferences and autonomy are involved.
8. **Limited Evidence:** For certain conditions or age groups, the evidence for the effectiveness and safety of medications may be limited.

It is crucial for parents, caregivers, and healthcare providers to have open and informed discussions about medication use in children. The decision to use medication should be based on a thorough evaluation of the child's specific condition, severity of symptoms, and individual needs. It is also essential to consider alternative treatments and lifestyle changes, and to engage in ongoing monitoring and communication to ensure the child's safety and well-being.

As with any medical intervention, the use of medication in children should be guided by experienced healthcare professionals, and the potential benefits and risks should be carefully considered to make informed decisions that support the child's health and overall development.

C. Integrative approaches to treatment

Integrative approaches to treatment involve combining complementary and alternative therapies with conventional medical treatments to address various health conditions. These approaches recognize the value of different healing modalities and aim to create a comprehensive and personalized treatment plan for the individual. Integrative approaches consider the whole person, including physical, emotional, social, and spiritual aspects of health. Here are some common integrative approaches to treatment:

1. **Complementary and Alternative Medicine (CAM):** CAM includes a wide range of therapies and practices, such as acupuncture,

chiropractic care, herbal medicine, meditation, yoga, massage therapy, and mindfulness techniques. These therapies can be used alongside conventional medical treatments to enhance overall well-being and manage symptoms.

2. Nutrition and Diet: Integrative medicine emphasizes the role of nutrition and diet in supporting health and healing. It may involve personalized dietary plans, nutritional supplements, and education on making healthy food choices.

3. Mind-Body Therapies: Mind-body therapies, such as meditation, guided imagery, relaxation techniques, and biofeedback, promote the connection between the mind and body, reducing stress and enhancing coping skills.

4. Exercise and Physical Activity: Regular exercise is an integral part of integrative approaches to treatment. Physical activity has numerous benefits for both physical and mental health, and it can complement medical treatments.

5. Psychosocial Support: Integrative approaches recognize the importance of psychosocial factors in health and healing. Counseling, psychotherapy, support groups, and other forms of psychosocial support may be included in treatment plans.

6. Lifestyle Modifications: Integrative medicine emphasizes lifestyle changes, such as getting adequate sleep, managing stress, reducing exposure to toxins, and fostering healthy relationships.

7. Herbal and Nutritional Supplements: Some integrative treatments may include the use of herbal remedies and nutritional supplements to support the body's natural healing processes.

8. Traditional Healing Systems: Integrative approaches may draw from traditional healing systems, such as Traditional Chinese Medicine (TCM) or Ayurveda, to address health imbalances.

9. Energy Medicine: Energy-based therapies, such as Reiki or Healing Touch, are used to promote energetic balance and support the body's natural healing abilities.

10. Patient-Centered Care: Integrative medicine places a strong emphasis on patient-centered care, taking into account the individual's preferences, beliefs, and goals in developing the treatment plan.

Integrative approaches to treatment recognize that each person is unique and that healing requires a holistic and individualized approach. The goal is to combine the best of both conventional and complementary therapies to optimize health outcomes and improve the overall well-being of the individual. It is important for individuals to work closely with healthcare professionals who are experienced in integrative medicine to develop a tailored treatment plan that meets their specific needs and preferences.

X. Nurturing Resilience and Emotional Well-being

A. The role of physical activity and a healthy lifestyle

Physical activity and a healthy lifestyle play a crucial role in promoting overall well-being and preventing various health conditions. They have a significant impact on both physical and mental health, and incorporating regular exercise and healthy habits into one's life can lead to numerous benefits. Here are some key roles of physical activity and a healthy lifestyle:

1. Physical Health:

- **Cardiovascular Health:** Regular physical activity improves cardiovascular health, reducing the risk of heart disease, hypertension, and stroke.
- **Weight Management:** Maintaining a healthy weight through regular exercise and a balanced diet helps prevent obesity and related health issues.
- **Bone Health:** Weight-bearing exercises, such as walking and resistance training, support bone health and reduce the risk of osteoporosis.
- **Immune Function:** Regular physical activity boosts the immune system, making the body more resilient to infections and illnesses.
- **Chronic Disease Prevention:** A healthy lifestyle reduces the risk of chronic conditions, such as type 2 diabetes and certain types of cancer.

2. Mental Health:

- **Stress Reduction:** Physical activity helps reduce stress and promotes relaxation, leading to improved mental well-being.

- **Mood Enhancement:** Exercise triggers the release of endorphins, the "feel-good" chemicals in the brain, which can enhance mood and reduce symptoms of anxiety and depression.
- **Cognitive Function:** Regular physical activity is associated with better cognitive function, memory, and attention.
- **Sleep Quality:** A healthy lifestyle, including regular exercise, promotes better sleep quality and duration.

3. Energy and Vitality:

- **Increased Energy Levels:** Regular physical activity boosts energy levels and reduces feelings of fatigue.
- **Improved Productivity:** A healthy lifestyle can lead to improved focus, productivity, and overall performance in daily activities.

4. Social Interaction:

- **Opportunities for Socialization:** Participating in group activities or sports provides opportunities for social interaction and fosters a sense of community.

5. Longevity and Quality of Life:

- **Longevity:** Regular physical activity and a healthy lifestyle are associated with increased life expectancy.
- **Enhanced Quality of Life:** Maintaining good physical and mental health through a healthy lifestyle enhances overall quality of life and well-being.

6. Self-Esteem and Confidence:

- **Self-Esteem:** Achieving fitness goals and adopting healthy habits can boost self-esteem and self-confidence.
- **Positive Body Image:** Regular physical activity and a focus on overall health contribute to a positive body image.

7. Disease Management:

- **Management of Chronic Conditions:** Physical activity and healthy habits can complement medical treatments in managing chronic health conditions.

8. Role Modeling: Leading a healthy lifestyle can positively influence family members and peers, promoting healthier habits in the community.

It is essential to find physical activities that one enjoys to maintain consistency and sustainability. Combining aerobic exercises, strength training, flexibility exercises, and relaxation techniques can provide a well-rounded approach to physical activity. Adopting a healthy lifestyle also involves balanced nutrition, hydration, adequate sleep, and managing stress. Consulting with healthcare professionals and seeking support from friends, family, or health coaches can be beneficial in developing and maintaining a personalized plan for a healthy lifestyle.

B. Fostering positive relationships and social support

Fostering positive relationships and social support is essential for overall well-being and mental health. Human beings are social creatures, and meaningful connections with others contribute significantly to happiness, resilience, and emotional health. Here are some key aspects of fostering positive relationships and social support:

1. Building Meaningful Connections:

- Invest time and effort in building and maintaining meaningful relationships with family, friends, colleagues, and community members.
- Engage in activities and groups that align with your interests and values to meet like-minded individuals.

2. Active Communication:

- Practice active listening and empathetic communication when interacting with others.
- Express gratitude and appreciation for the support and kindness received from friends and loved ones.

3. Nurturing Supportive Friendships:

- Cultivate friendships based on mutual respect, trust, and understanding.
- Be available to provide support and lend a listening ear to friends in times of need.

4. Seeking and Offering Help:

- Don't hesitate to ask for help when needed, as it strengthens the bonds with others and allows them to contribute positively to your well-being.
- Offer your help and support to others when they require assistance, as helping others can be emotionally rewarding and strengthens social bonds.

5. Participating in Social Activities:

- Engage in social activities and events, such as clubs, classes, sports, or community gatherings.
- Volunteering and engaging in community service activities can also foster a sense of belonging and social connectedness.

6. Boundaries and Respect:

- Establish healthy boundaries in relationships to maintain emotional well-being.
- Treat others with respect, kindness, and understanding to

create a supportive and positive social environment.

7. Online and Offline Connections:

- Balance online and offline interactions, as online connections can provide support but may not substitute for in-person relationships.

8. Support During Difficult Times:

- Seek social support during challenging times, as sharing feelings and experiences with trusted individuals can alleviate stress and provide comfort.

9. Celebrating Achievements Together:

- Share achievements and successes with loved ones, celebrating each other's accomplishments.

10. Being a Positive Influence:

- Strive to be a positive influence on others by offering encouragement, support, and positivity.

11. Joining Supportive Groups:

- Seek out support groups or communities centered around shared experiences or interests to find individuals who can relate to your journey and provide understanding.

Positive relationships and social support can act as a buffer during times of stress and adversity. They provide emotional validation, a sense of belonging, and can help individuals cope with life's challenges. Cultivating and nurturing these connections is a continuous process that requires effort, but the rewards in terms of happiness, emotional well-being, and resilience are invaluable.

C. Teaching resilience-building skills in children

Teaching resilience-building skills in children is crucial for their emotional well-being and ability to cope with life's challenges. Resilience enables children to bounce back from setbacks, adapt to changes, and develop a positive outlook on life. Here are some effective strategies for teaching resilience-building skills to children:

1. Model Resilience:

- Children learn by observing their parents, caregivers, and teachers. Model resilience in your own life by demonstrating problem-solving, positive coping strategies, and a growth mindset in the face of difficulties.

2. Foster a Supportive Environment:

- Create a safe and supportive environment where children feel comfortable expressing their feelings and seeking help when needed.

3. Encourage Emotional Expression:

- Teach children to identify and express their emotions in healthy ways. Encourage them to talk about their feelings, whether positive or negative.

4. Develop Problem-Solving Skills:

- Help children develop problem-solving skills by encouraging them to think critically and find solutions to everyday challenges.

5. Build Self-Esteem:

- Praise children for their efforts and achievements, which helps build their self-esteem and confidence.

6. Teach Coping Strategies:

- Teach children various coping strategies, such as deep breathing, mindfulness, or engaging in enjoyable activities, to manage stress and anxiety.

7. Emphasize Growth Mindset:

- Foster a growth mindset by encouraging children to view challenges as opportunities for learning and growth rather than failures.

8. Encourage Perseverance:

- Encourage children to persevere through difficult tasks and setbacks, reinforcing the importance of effort and persistence.

9. Support Social Connections:

- Help children develop and maintain positive social connections with peers, as social support is a crucial factor in building resilience.

10. Focus on Gratitude:

- Teach children to practice gratitude by identifying things they are thankful for, which can foster a positive outlook on life.

11. Promote Healthy Habits:

- Encourage regular physical activity, proper nutrition, and adequate sleep, as these contribute to overall well-being and resilience.

12. Teach Stress Management:

- Help children recognize signs of stress and teach them relaxation techniques, such as deep breathing or progressive muscle relaxation.

13. Foster Problem-Focused Coping:

- Encourage children to approach challenges with a problem-focused coping style, seeking solutions and taking positive actions.

14. Provide Opportunities for Mastery:

- Offer children opportunities to develop and master new skills, which can enhance their sense of competence and self-efficacy.

15. Encourage a Sense of Purpose:

- Help children discover their passions and interests, encouraging a sense of purpose and meaning in their lives.

Remember that building resilience is a process that takes time and practice. Be patient and supportive as children develop these skills, and celebrate their progress along the way. By teaching resilience-building skills, you are equipping children with valuable tools that will serve them well throughout their lives.

XI. Prevention Strategies

A. Early intervention and mental health screening programs

Early intervention and mental health screening programs are essential components of a comprehensive approach to promoting mental health and well-being, especially in children and adolescents. These programs aim to identify and address mental health issues early, before they become more severe and have a significant impact on an individual's life. Here's an overview of the importance and benefits of early intervention and mental health screening programs:

Importance of Early Intervention:

1. **Prevention of Escalation:** Early intervention can prevent mild mental health concerns from escalating into more severe and chronic conditions. Addressing issues early can lead to better treatment outcomes.
2. **Reduced Stigma:** Early intervention helps reduce the stigma associated with mental health issues by promoting open conversations and awareness.
3. **Promotion of Healthy Coping Strategies:** Early intervention allows individuals to learn and develop healthy coping strategies, which can enhance their resilience and ability to manage stress.
4. **Improved Academic and Social Outcomes:** Addressing mental health concerns early can positively impact academic performance, social relationships, and overall quality of life.
5. **Support for Families:** Early intervention programs often involve support and resources for families, empowering them to navigate mental health challenges effectively.

Benefits of Mental Health Screening Programs:

1. **Early Identification:** Screening programs identify mental

health concerns early, allowing for timely intervention and support.

2. **Preventive Measures:** Screening can identify risk factors and early signs of mental health issues, enabling preventive measures to be implemented.

3. **Improved Access to Services:** Screening programs help individuals and families connect with appropriate mental health services and resources.

4. **Increased Awareness:** Screening programs raise awareness about mental health and the importance of early intervention in the community.

5. **Data Collection:** Screening programs provide valuable data on mental health trends and needs, assisting in the development of targeted interventions.

Implementation Challenges and Considerations:

1. **Cultural Sensitivity:** Mental health screening programs should be culturally sensitive and consider the unique needs and perspectives of diverse communities.

2. **Confidentiality and Privacy:** Ensuring confidentiality and privacy is essential in mental health screening to protect individuals' rights and encourage participation.

3. **Effective Communication:** Clear communication is crucial in explaining the purpose and benefits of screening to individuals and families.

4. **Resource Allocation:** Adequate resources and funding are necessary for the successful implementation and sustainability of screening programs.

5. **Collaboration:** Collaboration between healthcare providers, schools, community organizations, and mental health professionals is key to the success of screening initiatives.

Early intervention and mental health screening programs are instrumental in promoting mental health, preventing the worsening of mental health conditions, and improving overall well-being. By addressing mental health concerns early, individuals can receive the support and resources they need to lead healthier and more fulfilling lives.

B. Raising awareness of childhood depression and reducing stigma

Raising awareness of childhood depression and reducing stigma are crucial steps in promoting early identification and access to appropriate support and treatment for affected children. Here are some strategies to achieve these goals:

1. Education and Information Dissemination:

- Educate parents, caregivers, teachers, and the general public about childhood depression, its signs, symptoms, and prevalence.
- Share accurate information through workshops, seminars, online resources, and educational materials.

2. Encourage Open Conversations:

- Promote open and non-judgmental conversations about mental health, including childhood depression.
- Encourage individuals to share their experiences and stories to reduce the stigma associated with seeking help.

3. Use Media Effectively:

- Utilize various media channels to raise awareness about childhood depression and mental health.
- Collaborate with media outlets to spread positive and accurate portrayals of mental health issues.

4. Schools and Education Programs:

- Introduce mental health education in schools to increase students' awareness and understanding.
- Train teachers and school staff to recognize signs of childhood depression and provide appropriate support.

5. Community Events and Campaigns:

- Organize community events and campaigns to promote mental health awareness and reduce stigma.
- Involve local organizations and leaders to reach a broader audience.

6. Collaborate with Mental Health Professionals:

- Collaborate with mental health professionals to provide accurate information and resources.
- Encourage mental health professionals to actively engage in community awareness initiatives.

7. Engage Youth:

- Involve young people in awareness campaigns and initiatives to make the messages more relatable and impactful.
- Empower youth to become advocates for mental health and challenge stigma among their peers.

8. Share Success Stories:

- Share success stories of individuals who sought help for childhood depression and recovered, demonstrating that seeking support is a positive and empowering step.

9. Address Cultural and Social Barriers:

- Be sensitive to cultural beliefs and practices that may affect how childhood depression is perceived.

- Address social norms that discourage seeking help for mental health issues.

10. Provide Accessible Resources:

- Make mental health resources, helplines, and support services easily accessible and widely available.
- Ensure that information is available in different languages and formats to reach diverse populations.

11. Train Healthcare Providers:

- Provide training to healthcare providers on identifying and treating childhood depression.
- Encourage healthcare providers to approach mental health with empathy and understanding.

12. Advocate for Policy Changes:

- Advocate for policies that support mental health awareness and reduce stigma in schools, workplaces, and healthcare settings.

By raising awareness and reducing stigma surrounding childhood depression, we can create a more supportive and understanding environment for affected children and their families. Early identification and intervention are vital in ensuring that children receive the help they need to thrive and lead healthier lives.

C. Collaborating with schools, communities, and healthcare professionals

Collaborating with schools, communities, and healthcare professionals is a powerful approach to promoting mental health awareness, early intervention, and comprehensive support for children facing depression. Each of these stakeholders plays a unique role in a child's life, and their combined efforts can create a supportive and integrated system. Here are ways to foster collaboration:

1. Mental Health Education in Schools:

- Collaborate with schools to incorporate mental health education and awareness programs into the curriculum.
- Train teachers and school staff to recognize signs of childhood depression and provide appropriate support.

2. School-Based Screening and Referral Programs:

- Work with schools and healthcare professionals to implement mental health screening programs for early identification of at-risk children.
- Establish referral pathways to connect children in need with appropriate mental health services.

3. Parent and Caregiver Engagement:

- Engage parents and caregivers through workshops and support groups to raise awareness of childhood depression and available resources.
- Foster open communication between schools, parents, and mental health professionals to provide holistic support to children.

4. Community Awareness Events and Initiatives:

- Organize community events and campaigns to promote mental health awareness, reduce stigma, and provide information about childhood depression.
- Partner with community organizations, local businesses, and religious institutions to reach a broader audience.

5. Healthcare Provider Training:

- Provide training to healthcare professionals, including pediatricians and family doctors, on recognizing and addressing childhood depression.
- Collaborate with healthcare providers to ensure a seamless referral process to specialized mental health services.

6. Integrated Care Models:

- Develop integrated care models that involve collaboration between schools, mental health professionals, and primary healthcare providers.
- Ensure that information is shared appropriately and that care is coordinated across different settings.

7. Telehealth and Virtual Platforms:

- Utilize telehealth and virtual platforms to facilitate communication and collaboration between schools, communities, and healthcare professionals.
- Offer virtual counseling and support services for children and families who may face barriers to in-person care.

8. Supportive School Environment:

- Advocate for a supportive school environment that promotes mental health and well-being.
- Encourage schools to implement anti-bullying programs and foster a culture of empathy and inclusivity.

9. Research and Data Sharing:

- Collaborate on research initiatives to understand the prevalence and impact of childhood depression in the community.

- Share data and insights to inform evidence-based interventions and policies.

10. Advocacy for Mental Health Services:

- Advocate for increased funding and resources for mental health services in schools and communities.
- Raise awareness about the importance of mental health in policy discussions and community forums.

By working together, schools, communities, and healthcare professionals can create a comprehensive support system that addresses childhood depression holistically. The collective effort can lead to earlier identification, timely intervention, and improved outcomes for children's mental health and well-being.

XII. Real-life Success Stories

A. Inspirational stories of children who have overcome depression

Inspiring stories of children who have overcome depression serve as powerful reminders of resilience and the potential for recovery. While each individual's journey is unique, these stories can provide hope and encouragement to others facing similar challenges. Here are a few examples of such stories:

1. **Emma's Triumph:** Emma, a 12-year-old girl, struggled with depression due to bullying at school. With the support of her parents and teachers, she sought counseling and began participating in self-defense classes to boost her confidence. Gradually, Emma learned to stand up for herself and found a passion for martial arts. Through her determination and newfound skills, she not only overcame depression but also became an advocate against bullying in her school, inspiring others to find their strength.

2. **Alex's Art Therapy:** Alex, a 10-year-old boy, experienced depression and anxiety following the loss of his parent. Traditional talk therapy did not seem to help him much. However, when he discovered art therapy, his life changed. Expressing his emotions through art allowed Alex to process his grief and find healing. His artwork became a form of self-expression and a source of strength. Today, Alex shares his art with others, showing that creativity can be a powerful tool for healing.

3. **Jake's Journey to Self-Discovery:** Jake, a 14-year-old struggling with depression and feelings of isolation, discovered the therapeutic benefits of nature and outdoor activities. He joined a local hiking group and began spending time in nature regularly. The calming effect of the natural surroundings and

the support of his newfound friends helped Jake gain perspective and cope with his emotions. His story shows how finding solace in nature can positively impact mental health.

4. **Mia's Mindfulness Practice:** Mia, an 8-year-old girl, experienced anxiety and low self-esteem, leading to depression. Her parents introduced her to mindfulness exercises and meditation techniques. Mia learned to be present in the moment and accept her thoughts and feelings without judgment. As she practiced mindfulness regularly, her anxiety reduced, and she became more self-assured. Mia's journey exemplifies the power of mindfulness in improving mental well-being.

5. **Ryan's Resilience through Sports:** Ryan, a 16-year-old boy, faced depression due to academic pressure and personal struggles. Engaging in sports, particularly running, became an outlet for him. Through running, he found a sense of accomplishment and purpose. As Ryan improved his physical health, he also noticed positive changes in his mental health. He now competes in marathons and shares his story to inspire others to find their passions.

These stories illustrate the diverse paths to overcoming depression, emphasizing that there is no one-size-fits-all approach to healing. The common threads among these stories are the unwavering support of family, friends, and professionals, and the children's courage to explore different coping strategies until they found what worked best for them. These examples demonstrate that recovery is possible and that with the right support and determination, children can rise above depression and reclaim their joy and resilience.

B. Insights from parents, therapists, and experts

Insights from parents, therapists, and experts are invaluable in understanding childhood depression, its impact, and effective ways to support children who experience it. Here are some key insights from these perspectives:

From Parents:

1. Early Signs Awareness: Parents may notice subtle changes in their child's behavior or mood that could be early signs of depression. Being attentive to these signs can facilitate early intervention.
2. Open Communication: Maintaining open and non-judgmental communication with their child allows parents to better understand their feelings and experiences.
3. Seeking Professional Help: Parents emphasize the importance of seeking help from mental health professionals when they observe concerning symptoms in their child, rather than dismissing them as "just a phase."
4. Supportive Environment: Creating a supportive and safe home environment helps children feel comfortable sharing their emotions and seeking help if needed.
5. Patience and Understanding: Parents stress the importance of patience and understanding while their child navigates through the challenges of depression.

From Therapists:

1. Holistic Approach: Therapists emphasize the need for a holistic approach to treating childhood depression, addressing emotional, psychological, and environmental factors.
2. Tailored Interventions: Effective interventions should be tailored to each child's unique needs and circumstances.
3. Family Involvement: Family involvement is crucial in the treatment process, as it supports the child's healing and helps in maintaining progress outside of therapy sessions.
4. Building Coping Skills: Therapists work on building coping

skills and resilience in children to equip them with tools to manage emotional challenges effectively.

5. Creating Trusting Relationships: Establishing a trusting and empathetic therapeutic relationship with the child is key to facilitating their healing and growth.

From Experts:

1. Early Intervention Impact: Experts stress the significance of early intervention in childhood depression to prevent long-term adverse effects on a child's development.
2. Stigma Reduction: Reducing stigma around mental health issues is essential to encourage help-seeking behavior in children and their families.
3. Multidisciplinary Collaboration: Collaborative efforts involving schools, communities, healthcare providers, and mental health professionals are critical in addressing childhood depression comprehensively.
4. Preventive Measures: Experts advocate for incorporating mental health education and coping skills training in school curricula to promote mental well-being and prevent depression.
5. Building Resilience: Fostering resilience in children through various activities and support systems can improve their ability to cope with life's challenges.

Overall, the insights from parents, therapists, and experts highlight the importance of early detection, a supportive environment, and individualized care to effectively address childhood depression. Collaborative efforts and a comprehensive approach that considers the child's whole ecosystem are key to helping children overcome depression and thrive in their lives.

XIII. Conclusion

A. Recapitulation of the importance of addressing childhood depression: Addressing childhood depression is of utmost importance due to the following reasons:

1. **Early Intervention for Better Outcomes:** Early identification and intervention can significantly improve a child's well-being and prevent the condition from becoming chronic or more severe later in life.

2. **Healthy Emotional Development:** By addressing depression, we can support children in developing emotionally, enabling them to build healthy relationships and cope with life's challenges.

3. **Academic Success and Learning:** Treating depression can improve a child's concentration, motivation, and engagement in learning, leading to better academic performance and educational achievements.

4. **Preventing Social Isolation:** Addressing depression helps children maintain social connections and friendships, reducing feelings of loneliness and isolation.

5. **Reducing Long-term Impact:** Untreated childhood depression can have long-term consequences on mental health and overall well-being, underscoring the need for timely intervention.

6. **Promoting Resilience:** By providing support and effective coping strategies, we empower children to build resilience, enabling them to face life's difficulties with strength and adaptability.

7. **Positive Family Dynamics:** Addressing childhood depression can improve family relationships, communication, and understanding, fostering a supportive and nurturing

environment.

8. **Preventing Suicidal Risk:** Depression is associated with an increased risk of self-harm and suicidal thoughts. Addressing it promptly reduces this risk and ensures the child's safety.

9. **Reducing Stigma:** By openly discussing childhood depression, we can reduce the stigma surrounding mental health, encouraging children and families to seek help without shame or judgment.

10. **Empowering the Next Generation:** By addressing childhood depression, we invest in the mental health and well-being of future generations, fostering a healthier and more resilient society.

Addressing childhood depression requires a collaborative effort involving parents, caregivers, educators, and mental health professionals. It is through awareness, understanding, and compassion that we can create an environment where children feel safe, supported, and empowered to overcome depression and thrive in their lives.

B. Empowering readers with knowledge and tools to support children's mental health:

Empowering readers with knowledge and tools to support children's mental health is a crucial aspect of the book. By providing practical information and strategies, the book aims to equip parents, caregivers, educators, and anyone involved in a child's life with the necessary tools to foster positive mental health in children. Here are some key ways the book can achieve this:

1. **Understanding Childhood Depression:** The book will provide readers with a comprehensive understanding of childhood depression, including its causes, signs, and symptoms. This knowledge will help them recognize when a child may be struggling with depression.

2. **Promoting Mental Health Awareness:** By raising awareness

about childhood mental health, the book will help readers recognize the importance of prioritizing a child's emotional well-being.

3. **Effective Communication:** The book will emphasize the significance of open and effective communication with children. It will offer guidance on how to talk to children about their feelings and emotions in a supportive and non-judgmental manner.

4. **Identifying Supportive Resources:** The book will guide readers in finding appropriate mental health resources, such as mental health professionals, support groups, and online resources, that can assist them in supporting children with depression.

5. **Building Resilience:** The book will introduce readers to strategies and activities that promote resilience in children, helping them develop coping skills to navigate life's challenges.

6. **Implementing Positive Parenting Techniques:** The book will explore positive parenting practices that nurture a child's emotional well-being and foster a strong parent-child bond.

7. **Creating a Supportive Environment:** The book will offer practical advice on how to create a supportive and nurturing environment at home, in school, and in the community.

8. **Encouraging Self-Care:** Readers will be reminded of the importance of self-care for both themselves and the children they care for. It will emphasize that taking care of one's own mental health is essential in supporting others.

9. **Understanding Different Therapeutic Approaches:** The book will provide insights into various therapeutic approaches for childhood depression, helping readers understand the available treatment options and when to seek professional help.

10. **Promoting Well-being through Play:** The book may introduce readers to play-based interventions and activities

that can support a child's emotional expression and healing.

By arming readers with practical knowledge and effective tools, the book will enable them to create a supportive and empathetic environment for children struggling with depression. Empowered with this understanding, readers can play a vital role in helping children build emotional resilience, fostering their mental health, and guiding them toward a brighter and more emotionally balanced future.

C. Encouragement to seek professional help and maintain hope for a brighter future

In the book, a heartfelt encouragement to seek professional help and maintain hope for a brighter future is essential to instill confidence in readers and children facing depression. Here's how the book can convey this message:

1. **Normalize Seeking Help:** The book should emphasize that seeking professional help for childhood depression is a sign of strength and courage, not weakness. It can reassure readers that reaching out for support is a natural and positive step toward healing.

2. **Highlighting the Impact of Professional Support:** By sharing stories of children who have benefited from professional help, the book can illustrate the positive impact that therapy and counseling can have on a child's mental health and overall well-being.

3. **Promoting a Collaborative Approach:** Encourage readers to work collaboratively with mental health professionals, educators, and other caregivers to create a holistic support network for the child. Stress the importance of open communication and shared goals.

4. **Expressing Empathy and Understanding:** Throughout the book, use language that conveys empathy and understanding for the challenges faced by both the child and their caregivers.

This fosters a sense of connection and validation for their experiences.

5. **Focus on Progress and Growth:** Emphasize that the journey to recovery may have ups and downs, but with consistent effort and professional guidance, positive progress can be made. Highlight the potential for growth and learning throughout the process.

6. **Celebrating Small Victories:** Encourage readers to celebrate every small victory and improvement the child makes, no matter how minor. This cultivates a sense of hope and motivation for continued progress.

7. **Promote Self-Compassion:** Remind readers that healing from depression takes time, and setbacks are a natural part of the process. Encourage self-compassion for both the child and their caregivers.

8. **Inspire Hope with Success Stories:** Share inspiring success stories of individuals who have overcome childhood depression and gone on to lead fulfilling and meaningful lives. This can provide hope and inspiration to readers facing similar challenges.

9. **Stress the Importance of Patience:** Encourage readers to be patient and understanding throughout the healing journey. Assure them that with time, dedication, and professional guidance, positive changes can be achieved.

10. **Focus on a Brighter Future:** Throughout the book, maintain a hopeful tone, emphasizing that childhood depression is treatable, and with the right support, children can move toward a brighter and emotionally balanced future.

By consistently reinforcing the message of seeking professional help and maintaining hope, the book can empower readers to take proactive steps to support children's mental health and foster a positive outlook for their emotional well-being.

www.ingramcontent.com/pod-product-compliance
Lightning Source LLC
Chambersburg PA
CBHW021755150726
47989CB00004B/1672